Self-Diagnosis, Healing and Recovery

Learn to Read Symptoms and Start Treatments on Your Own

By: Allison McPhee

9781681275208

PUBLISHERS NOTES

Disclaimer – Speedy Publishing LLC

This publication is intended to provide helpful and informative material. It is not intended to diagnose, treat, cure, or prevent any health problem or condition, nor is intended to replace the advice of a physician. No action should be taken solely on the contents of this book. Always consult your physician or qualified health-care professional on any matters regarding your health and before adopting any suggestions in this book or drawing inferences from it.

The author and publisher specifically disclaim all responsibility for any liability, loss or risk, personal or otherwise, which is incurred as a consequence, directly or indirectly, from the use or application of any contents of this book.

Any and all product names referenced within this book are the trademarks of their respective owners. None of these owners have sponsored, authorized, endorsed, or approved this book.

Always read all information provided by the manufacturers' product labels before using their products. The author and publisher are not responsible for claims made by manufacturers.

This book was originally printed before 2014. This is an adapted reprint by Speedy Publishing LLC with newly updated content designed to help readers with much more accurate and timely information and data.

Speedy Publishing LLC

40 E Main Street, Newark, Delaware, 19711

Contact Us: 1-888-248-4521

Website: http://www.speedypublishing.co

REPRINTED Paperback Edition: 9781681275208:

Manufactured in the United States of America

Dedication

This book is dedicated to Anthony. You are my prince charming.

TABLE OF CONTENTS

Chapter 1- Alternative Medicine in History

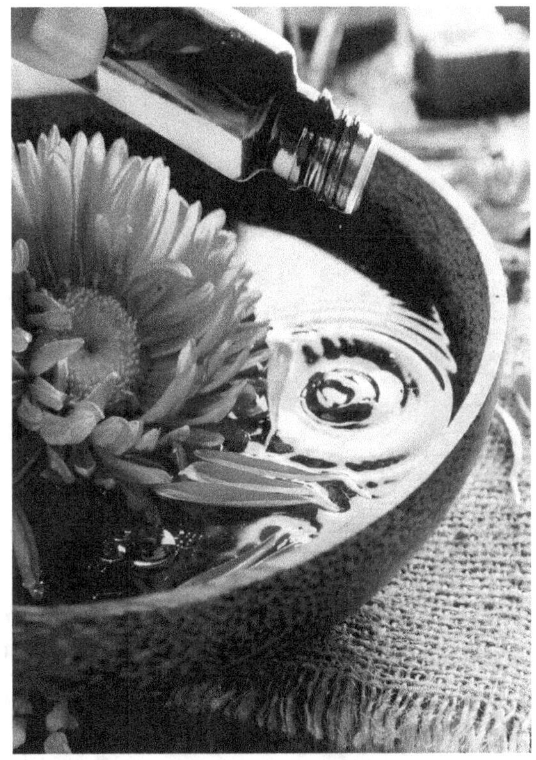

When most people get sick, they look to conventional methods of medical treatment for relief and healing. There are alternative methods to treatment that are becoming increasingly popular.

What treatments are considered "conventional?" Prescription medication, traditional surgery, and computerized scientific testing are three examples of conventional medicine. Most physicians support conventional medicine in their practices, so when seeing a doctor, it is highly likely you will be advised to follow conventional medical advice.

Self-Diagnosis, Healing and Recovery
The decision to use conventional medicine should be made by the patient and doctor on a case by case basis. An alteration to the type of treatment is sometimes all that is needed to feel better.

Alternative treatments include:

•Herbal remedies

•Massage

•Meditation

•Acupuncture

•Many more!

Patients will often find themselves turning to alternative methods of treatment when conventional methods are ineffective or a medical problem has been deemed untreatable. Alternative treatments are designed to not only aid in pain relief, but also reduce stress and tension that can worsen chronic pain.

Alternative methods of treatment focus on the whole person; body and soul. Convention methods strictly focus on the physical problems alone. For alternative methods to be effective, the patient must be motivated and believe in the alternative treatment's ability to work.

Of course, any serious, life-threatening health problem should blend conventional and alternative methods for a comprehensive approach. Be sure to consult with your doctor to avoid complications. If planned well, you can take advantage of best of both types of medicine for a life that is comfortable and enjoyable.

A Look into the Past

Thousands of years ago, all medicine was "alternative medicine." Before modern science, healers would consider the full picture - emotional, physical, and spiritual – before healing a sick person.

This is one of the main differences between modern conventional medicine and alternative medicine. Alternative medicine does not look for the instant cure for the physical problem, rather is looks more at a long-term solution that includes the whole self.

Just a few centuries ago in Europe there were two types of healers; folk healers that used old tried-and-true methods, and professional physicians. The lower classes did not have the money to pay for the professional physicians, but they used the folk healers and it worked.

In North America, philosophy and religion were often used to help folk healers provide holistic treatments.

The conventional medicine that we have today has evolved from the days of folk healers and alternative medicine. Many conventional physician support different types of holistic treatments in the overall wellness plan for their patients. The reason that alternative medicine has stood the test of time is because it works!

Ancient Chinese Medicine

Traditional Chinese medicine (TCM) includes acupuncture, Qigong, herbal treatments, deep massage, and more. More than 25% of the world's population practices TCM.

Several reputable groups, such as the World Health Organization and the National Institute of Health, find traditional Chinese medicine to be a viable alternative to contemporary medicine.

Many parts of TCM began well over 3,000 years ago in China. The focus of TCM is Qi (pronounced "Chee"), which is the body's energy that connects it to the world around us. It is believed that all disorders and bodily problems are caused by the misalignment of Qi. Acupuncture is one of the most widely recognized methods of bringing the Qi into alignment.

Herbal remedies are popular in traditional Chinese medicine. They are used to relax and calm the patient's emotions to avoid depression, and provide a more positive outlook on the illness. This helps tremendously in the healing process. Ginseng and herbal green tea are the most popular herbal remedies in China.

Exercise, mainly Qigong (pronounce "Chee Kung"), is also an important part of traditional Chinese medicine. Qigong involves posture, meditation, and slow, calculated body movements.

Tibetan Medicine

Tibetan Medicine is almost solely based on herbal remedies, and has been around for over 2,500 years. It is called "gSoba Rig-pa". Tibetans mostly live in India because they have been in exile since the late 1950's. They practice Tibetan Buddhism.

There is a Tibetan Medical Institute in Northern India, where doctors studying Tibetan medicine attend for 7 years before earning a degree.

The underlying belief in Tibetan medicine is that all illnesses are caused by poisonous thinking which include dread, denial, and want. This concept ties to the principles of Buddhist philosophy.

The three poisonous thoughts are believed to be caused by poor diet, inappropriate behavior, and the imbalance of time and season. This concept is more complicated than this, but this simplification will give a general sense of it.

Cures are linked to all systems of the body working together. The elimination of sweat, feces and urine contributes to this harmony.

Similar to the Chinese "Qi", the Tibetans have the Rlung, which is the overall life force that connects us to the universe. Rlung has five types:

1. Centered in the brain. Life grasping – controls breathing, intellect, sneezing and swallowing.

2. Centered in the chest. Upward moving – controls verbal ability and stamina.

3. Centered in the heart. All pervading – controls all movement like that of the orifices of the body and walking.

4. Centered in the stomach. Fire accompanying – controls digestion and metabolism.

5. Centered in the rectum. Downward cleansing – controls everything that is expelled from the body, such as babies, menstrual blood or semen.

Tibetan medicine usually handles sickness diagnosis by analysis of the tongue and urine. The spiritual element is also at play in

Tibetan medicine, with much attention spent focusing on the type and temperament of spirits in the body.

What is The Native American Medicine?

North American Indian tribes have been practicing medicine for what some claim to be over 40,000 years. The medical information and techniques are handed down from generation to generation; ensure the longevity of the practice.

Some remedies are tribe-specific, although all tribal medicine is called Native American Medicine, collectively. Native Americans believe that man is one with nature and that the elements provide strength and can cure disease.

It is fascinating to note that at the same time that Native American medicine was being practiced in North America, Traditional Chinese Medicine was being practiced a half a world away. Ayurveda (medicine practiced in India), was also practiced at this time, and will be covered next.

All of these traditional medical practices are based on the same fundamental belief that a person's lifestyle and environment should be taken into consideration before choosing a treatment path. There are subtle differences between the practices that are specific to the region.

Native American medicine recognizes a purification procedure involving herbal smoke before and after treatment. Treatments include the use of sage and cedar smoke to repel negative energy. Negative energy is considered the pain released by someone who is ill, or the pain that the healer takes on themselves from their patients. Therapeutic touch is used. Singing, chanting, drums and rattles accompany the healing during the session.

Ayurvedic Medicine

Ayurvedic Medicine is practiced in India, and focuses on natural healing. Practitioners believe that it is important for the body to be balanced, and all medicines are based on vegetables and minerals, with the active ingredients from plant alkaloids.

In Ayurvedic Medicine there is the belief that there are three elements in the body, called Kapha, Pitta, and Vata, that cause disease.

1. Kapha: This energy is caused by the lack of stabilizing the balance in the body. These are commonly called viruses by Westerners.

2. Pitta: This energy supports vision, temperature, hunger, thirst, intelligence, and happiness. When out of alignment, the outcomes include weight fluctuation, dehydration, depression, digestive issues, and apathy.

3. Vata: This energy keeps the overall balance between the earth, sky and world around us in check with ourselves. If it falls out of balance, sickness is invited in.

Disease is called Vyaadhi, and it is treated by focusing on the imbalance of elements.

Chapter 2- What Options Do You Have in Alternative Medicine?

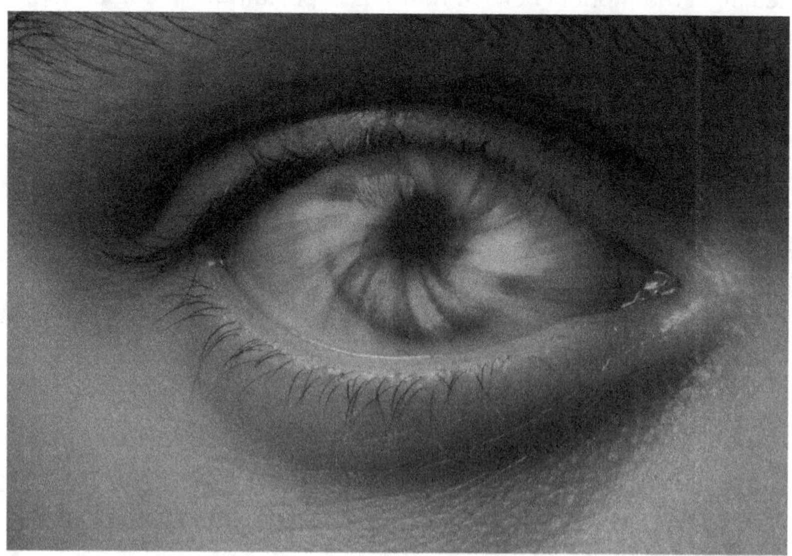

Homeopathy Treatments

Homeopathy is defined as an organic system of medicine that is based on three main ideas:

1. Like cures like

2. Minimal dosing

3. One time remedies

Alternative medicine traditionally has the least amount of "active" ingredient possible, with the concept of using one single remedy irregardless of how many symptoms are presenting. Homeopathy focuses on the least amount of treatments for better health.

There are several reasons why homeopathy is the second most popular form of medicine (after conventional medicine). The most popular reasons are:

• It is extremely natural and safe

• The results are permanent

• It is effective

• You can take most homeopathic medicines along with conventional medicine without side effects

• It is non-addictive

Homeopathy is a precise science, which is why it sometimes takes longer to find exactly the right medicine for your illness. Alternative medicine spends time asking questions about symptoms and the root cause of the illness in an effort to make a clear diagnosis for the problem, and treat it effectively.

Herbal Remedies

Nature provides many cures and treatments for ailments of all kinds. Each region has its own native plants that are used in alternative medicine.

When buying herbs for medicinal purposes, it is suggested that you use herbs from an herbal shop. Herb strength varies depending on the way in which they are grown, so until you are familiar with growing techniques for medicinal herbs, purchasing from a professional is recommended.

The following list provides herbal cures to common ailments:

•Acne and skin blemishes.

Wash your face and rub a clove of garlic that has been cut in half. Or, mix lavender with witch hazel at a 1:10 ratio. Tea tree oil can be substituted in place of the lavender.

•Anxiety and stress.

Lavender pure essential oil soaked onto a cotton cloth, heated, and folded into a compress. Apply to head or neck.

•Bruises and contusions.

Boil hyssop flowers and leaves into a tincture. Filter liquid, and soak a cotton compress. Apply to bruised area by applying pressure. The hyssop, heat and pressure combination will reduce the bruise.

•Burns.

Minor burns can be treated with comfrey or aloe juice. Simply rub aloe juice into burned area. Comfrey can be crushed into a fine powder, mixed with equal parts of melted beeswax, and added to vegetable oil. Simmer over low heat for 20 minutes, and then strain mixture.

•Warts.

Either use a cut piece of garlic, placed directly on the wart or, for a less odorous cure, try dandelion juice applied repeatedly throughout the day.

Herbal Teas

Allison McPhee

An age old remedy, herbal teas are used to soothe and relive pain and stress. Many teas are actually a tincture rather than a tea. A tincture is a thicker tea that is herb-dense and is infused instead of steeped.

The following list is a list of conditions and herbal tea remedies:

•Anemia.

Drink a tincture made from boiled stinging nettle leaves.

•Arthritis.

Drink a tincture of devil's claw, juniper, birch, or celery seed (not the type on your spice rack).

•Chemotherapy side effects.

Drink a tincture of Siberian ginseng root. It soothes the insides and relieves fatigue.

•Colic in babies.

Add less than 10 drops of dill and fennel tincture to their bottle.

•Constipation.

Drink a liter of rhubarb root per day.

•Cough.

Drink a tea made from garlic bulbs and ribwort leaves.

•Depression.

Drink a tincture daily made from the ground up oat plant and St. John's wart flowers.

•Fever.

Drink a hot tea made of lemon balm, yarrow, and ginger.

•Gas.

Drink a tea made of caraway, fennel, ginger, and peppermint.

•Flu symptoms.

Drink a tincture made of Echinacea, yarrow, and catnip.

Vitamins & Minerals

Taking a vitamin supplement is not a substitution for eating healthfully. However, it does serve as insurance to be certain that you are getting all of the vitamins and minerals that your body needs.

Vitamins are essential to the optimized functioning of your body. Without sufficient vitamins, for example, your blood will not clot. You need vitamins to fight colds, and boost your immune system.

It is best to take a homeopathic test to determine the vitamins that you need. This will avoid a dangerous overdose. Then you can take the vitamins you need individually, as needed, and avoid a multi-vitamin, which is chockfull of fillers. This method will save you money, too.

Bee Therapy (aka Apitherapy)

The practice of Apitherapy is the use of bee stings, bee pollen, propolis, royal jelly, and honey to treat a variety of ailments. While there has not been extensive testing in the scientific world to validate the claims of apitherapists, history proves that the treatments provide relief.

There are five honeybee products that are used in Apitherapy:

1. Venom: A practitioner will aid the patient in injecting or being stung by bees in the affected area. The venom is used to provide relief for conditions such as tendonitis, Multiple Sclerosis, and degenerative bone disease. It works because the venom is a natural anti-inflammatory which is more potent than others available to conventional medicine such as hydrocortisone. You must get tested to be certain that you are not allergic to beestings prior to exposing yourself to bee venom.

2. Pollen: A natural energy supplement that is also used as a seasonal allergy aid. It is also believed to slow down the development of wrinkles.

3. Raw Honey: A source of quick energy, raw honey is used for many cures. It can even be used as a salve on top of an open wound to avoid the spread of bacteria.

4. Royal Jelly: Is the milky white substance that the worker bees produce to feed the queen. While unsubstantiated, this substance is used as a beauty aid and is believed to help lower cholesterol.

5. Propolis: Is the glue used to keep the hives together and make repairs. Propolis is made from the sap of poplar and conifer trees. It is used to make lip balm and salves, and is considered to be an antioxidant.

Iridology

Iridology is name for the practice of determining a person's toxicity based on the color of their iris. This concept goes back to Sweden and Hungary where physicians used it to gauge disease in their patients.

For centuries, famous physicians and scientists, all the way back to the Greek physician Hippocrates; have found the people with injuries get black marks across the iris of their eye. These marks later disappear as the person's ailments heal.

In today's world, iridology is used as a preventative measure to gauge if there is a change in a person's health. It is unfortunate that iridology cannot be used to identify a specific disease.

The way in which iridology is practiced today is that the colored part of the eye (the iris) is carefully photographed using a strong camera lens. It is painless, and it takes about an hour to complete. The photos are then enlarged, and a trained professional iridologist studies it for signs of possible illness.

Even conventional doctors use the eyes as an early warning sign of bad things going on inside of the body. This study is just the more focused analysis of the iris when looking for signs of degenerative health issues.

Neuro Linguistic Programming (NLP)

Neuro Linguistic Programming can be considered the power of positive thought and prayer. It is well documented throughout science and medicine that having a positive attitude, outlook, and having a positive support system surround you is one of the most effective alternative medicines available.

NLP is a method of programming your thoughts in order to be positive. This technique focuses on your sub-conscious and your dreams. It is imperative to truly believe that you can heal yourself for NLP to work.

How do you practice NLP? First, take a strategy that you know creates success in other areas of your life, and apply it to your healing process. You absolutely must have faith in your body's healing ability for this to work.

Chapter 3- Muscular and Skeletal Alternative Medicine

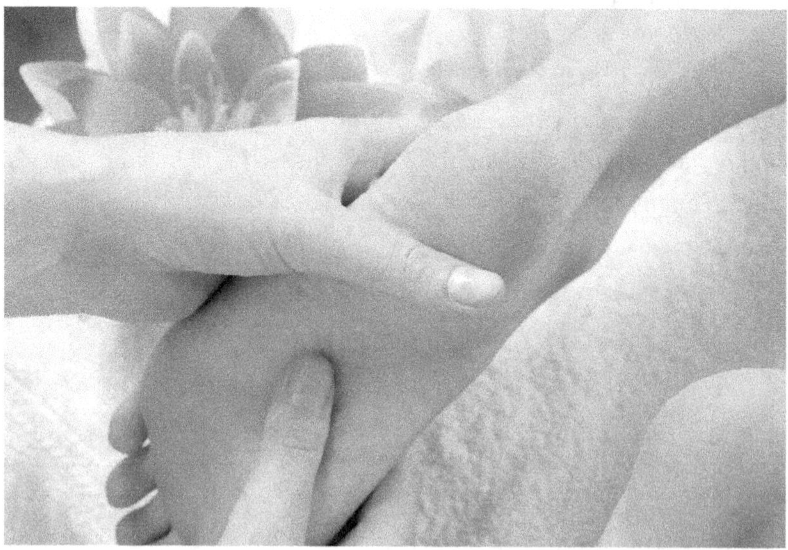

There are numerous other alternative treatments for the skeletal and muscular systems of the body. They include:

1.Kinesiology

Professionals test the various muscles throughout the body to determine areas that are not balanced properly, and then restore balance by using a variety of techniques.

2.Rolfing

Rolfing is the use of pressure to massage the connective tissue within the body. This allows for the body to be more flexible and be aligned properly. Rolfing will provide more energy and less anxiety.

3. Massage Therapy

Massage therapy is used to break up the knotted muscles, and to retrain the muscles. It works the ligaments, tendons, and soft tissue muscles. Massage therapy increases circulation and improves breathing.

4. Color therapy

Color therapy uses color and light to treat ailments. Often considered a complementary treatment, color therapy is used in addition to other treatment. There are seven colors that correspond to the wavelength centers of the body. Each color is matched with a region of the body.

5. Magnetic energy

The use of magnetic energy fields to, as magnetic therapists believe, to manipulate cells with magnetic energy. They also believe they can recharge cells. Magnetic energy can also increase blood flow that will then reduce scars on organs, provide migraine relief, and other reoccurring pain.

6. Craniosacral therapy (CST)

The craniosacral system is the membranes and fluid that envelopes the brain and spinal cord. By applying gentle pressure to the head, the rhythm of the craniosacral system can be evaluated and in some ways manipulated. This improves the flow and function of the central nervous system. This treatment is used in alternative medicine as a preventative measure. Professional craniosacral therapy practitioners believe they can locate and release energy cysts by unblocking them and realigning the neck.

Acupuncture

In acupuncture, thin needles are inserted into the skin to draw nerve stimulation at pinpointed locations around the body. Acupuncture is a Chinese medical procedure that involves Dao – the advocate for living in balance and moderation, with ying and yang – two life elements that are opposing forces that when balanced brings good health and happiness. Acupuncture brings relief of pain, aids respiratory illnesses, and relieves headaches and ulcers, among other physical issues. It also balances the qi life force.

Reiki

Reiki is the practice of transferring healing energy from the healer's hands to the ill person. This can be done hands-on and from a distance. The healer is believed to be full of universal energy. It is thought that the practitioner can use Reiki energy to alter the frequency of the aura. Healing is achieved first physically, then emotionally, and finally spiritually.

Crystals: A Tool for Healing

Crystals have long been associated with alternative healing. A crystal is created when crystalline is formed by minerals being arranged in a precise pattern. Quartz is the most popular crystal. The belief behind the use of crystals is that blocked energy will be released when the crystal is placed at specific points around the body.

CHAPTER 4- HOW TO DEVELOP THE RIGHT ENERGY FOR SELF-HEALING

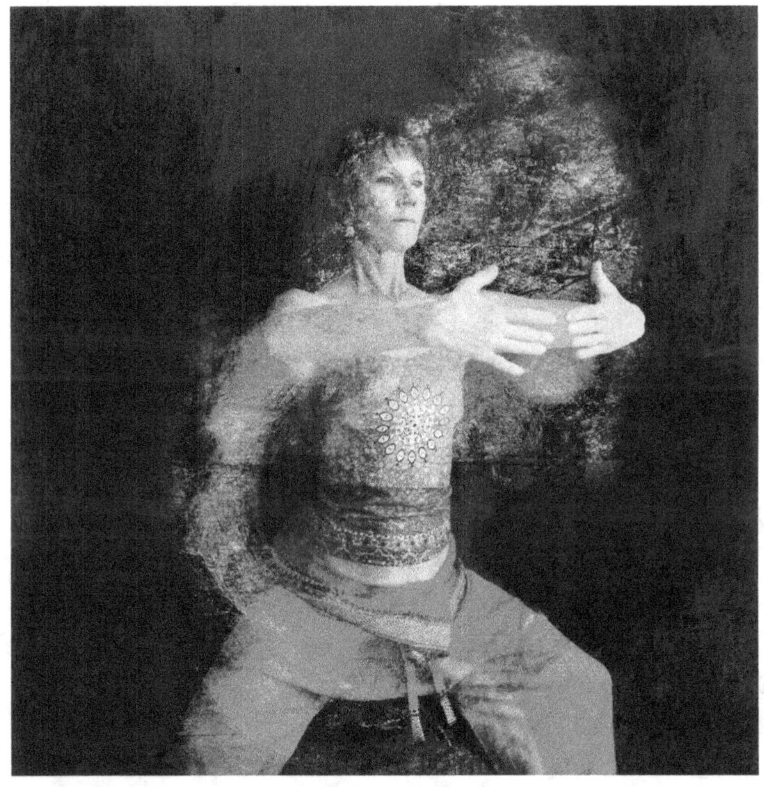

Energy development is important for self-healing. The reason is when you build your metabolic system you are improving your life sustaining. To build system however you must learn a few energy development practices in self-healing. Some of the basic practices are commonsense, since your body and mind needs exercise and proper nutrition to survive. When you do not take care of your body and mind, by ignoring its basic needs, you are only causing your body harm. You can focus on exercising the mind firstly to build your motivation to start healing your body.

Mind exercises in energy development and self-healing practices-in how it works: To begin mind exercises think about what it will take to encourage living cells to continue reproducing and replacing dying cells. After you turn 30, living cells slow its production and dying cells increase its production, which means your life is shorten. To promote living cells you will need to keep your brain active, focusing on positive things that will encourage you to take action.

How it Works

You have a few options in brain training, which includes writing, meditation, and accelerated practices and so on. Search the Internet to learn some of your options. Look for self-development practices that will lead you to discover what your brain needs to encourage your body to heal. When you research, you learn something new, which is a great exercise for your brain. With each piece of knowledge you take in, your brain will reward you with positive thinking that encourages energy.

When you research think of something about you that you want to change and then go online to find out information about this issue. When you learn something new about you, you can take steps to build energy and heal the body and mind.

You can practice meditation also to encourage energy and self-healing. In addition, when you meditate you explore the mind, learning something new about you. You develop new skills, new ideas and so on that encourage your brain to welcome rejuvenated energies. Into the bargain, when you cogitate you explore your mind, learning something new about you. This is a practice in subliminal exploring or learning.

You expand new credentials, new ideas and so on that propose your brain to congenial re-energized natural and positive energies.

This is the key points in exercising the brain that will benefit you and help you to see how you can heal the body and mind.

The Benefits of Energy Development and Self-Healing

Learning who you are is essential in discovering techniques to improve your overall life and health. Take time now to learn tactics you can use to learn more about you. Include meditation in your daily schedule to increase your pace at healing your body and mind.

Energy betterment is critical for self-assurance-healing. Some of the intrinsic practices we can use to benefit our life are based on our own innate understanding. Take time to explore subliminal learning to learn more about what you know, what skills you can develop and how connecting with your subconscious mind will benefit you. Your body and mind needs sporting and proper nutrition to survive. For this reason, you need to consider and devise a plan to focus on diet and exercise.

If you exercise the body you build muscles, healthy bones, joints, etc. and you also encourage living cells and the metabolic system to continue producing what you need to survive healthy. To learn more take some time to explore subliminal exploring in energy development and self-healing.

How Subliminal Exploring Helps

By exploring your subconscious mind you will learn something about you that you can use in your goal to energy development and self-healing. When you explore the subliminal mind you begin to challenge the mind, acquirements and learn something new about who you are. As you continue to explore you begin to mature, developing new skills, new thoughts or ideas that guides you to discover ways to build energy and heal the body and mind. Moreover, you give your brain the confidence it needs to open its arms to recharged power supplies of sources, or energies.

To understand how subliminal exploring in energy development and self-healing works, think of a battery that operates a vehicle. To keep this battery live and active you must supply it with water, charges, etc. to give it the energy to continue producing charge to operate your vehicle. If you fail to recharge your battery, or give it water when it needs it, the battery will soon stop working. Like this battery, your brain and body also needs water, nutrition, and recharging to continue producing its natural chemicals and substances.

To do this you would have to learn brain exercises that include subliminal exploring. When you practice subliminal or subconscious exploring, you work toward encouraging the mind to work in harmony with all aspects of the mind and body. This is the process of building energies, because your mind is getting the food it needs. That is your mind expects to learn and development. This is your intentions and you must encourage this process by upholding the law of nature, i.e. giving your mind and body proper food, exercise, relaxation and so on. Energy development is of great consequence for self-natural medicine. To build energy however you must think brain exercise, body exercise and nutrition.

Basic brain exercises include subliminal exploring, meditation, relaxation, natural practices, learning, and so on. You can benefit by practicing meditation daily to explore your subconscious mind. Some of the basic limited choice is built on our ability to use our commonsense. For instance, if you see a vehicle coming in your direction, you would naturally move out of the way rather than take the risk of the car hitting you. Well, as if your commonsense tells you to move out of the way of the oncoming vehicle, your mind also tells you when it is suffering. You experience stress and emotional charges that send you signal. This is when you want to feed your mind. In fact, if you feed your mind daily you would not have as many emotional charges or volume of stress. This is a great way to self-healing the body and mind, since when the mind is over consumed the body suffers gravely.

Body exercise – Now to encourage your mind, your body demands exercise. Keeping the bones, muscles and joints active will encourage mobility, energy and will inspire your mind to focus on energy development and self-healing continuously. This is because you are inspiring the metabolic system, nervous system, muscles, joints, living cells, and so to continue. When you learn to train your body and mind from exercise, meditation, subliminal exploring and other healthy practices will fall into place. Each day that you strive to reach your goal, you will find it easier to encourage energy development and self-healing of the body and mind.

How to Explore Your Inner Self

Reach inside your inner self and do some exploring to learn things you did not realize existed. Use the results to increase your energy and develop skills while working toward self-healing. Put your brain and mind to work by challenging your mind to find out whom you are and how you feel about yourself. Exploring the real person inside you to learn and grow from your findings. As you find who is inside you will be able to develop skills to help you build your energy and self-healing skills. Increase the brain confidence will give your mind energy. Give your brain and mind an awakening sense of energy. You will need to start by exploring your mind and discovering that exercise for the brain and body is essential to heal the soul.

The brain needs to exercise just as our bodies need exercise to keep it limber and giving full performance. Build your energy by exploring your mind for self-healing and giving it the exercise, it needs. Subliminal learning takes practice to help you to think positive and to replace the loss of bodily requirements that occur with age. By exercising your mind and body often you will new skills and notice a difference in your health. The brain and mind will build energy for self-healing with exercise. Giving your mind and brain exercise is like giving it food. We need food to build and maintain our bodies in order to have a healthy life. When you fail to exercise the brain, it slows the growing process, which only leads to poor health.

Learn to practice meditation by exploring the inner mind. Learn new skills and practice, how to relax with daily meditation to build energy development and self-healing skills. Meditation will give you skills to relax, relieve pain, and be successful with your true self. Learning and practicing to give the brain exercise will give you many new skills that you never imagined.

When we give the brain daily exercise, we can help prevent stress, heart disease and other signs of aging. Exercise with exploring the mind will give us a longer and happier life. Setting goals will provide exercise to the brain and mind by exploring yourself to finding whom you are and how to make changes to improve your energy development and self-healing goals.

Energize your brain and body with meditation to explore you. Energy will keep your bones, muscles, and brain active and healthy. Exercise will give inspiration to your joints, nervous system, and living cells to keep them active and encouraging them to keep going. This will provide you with the food and nutrition you and your body need to survive. Stay active and new skills and developments will come to you for reaching your goals to success.

Allison McPhee

You can find many different ways on how to development new skills by thinking positive, meditation, and exercise by taking some time out to researching the Internet.

Going online will help you find answers to all the questions you might have on how to improve your energy development and self-healing. To get started search for great products, programs and even educational courses that will guide you to energy development and self-healing. Look for the latest accelerated training courses. These courses guide you to relax and to learn through repetitive procedures. You learn quicker.

These are great self-development programs, which is something you need to encourage energy and self-healing. Some of the Neurofeedback programs online will benefit you in many ways. Take time to explore how you can learn to relax, which is a great start to energy development and self-healing. Boosting energy in meditation is possible by writing your feelings and emotions on paper.

Chapter 5- Better Energy Development for Better Self-Healing

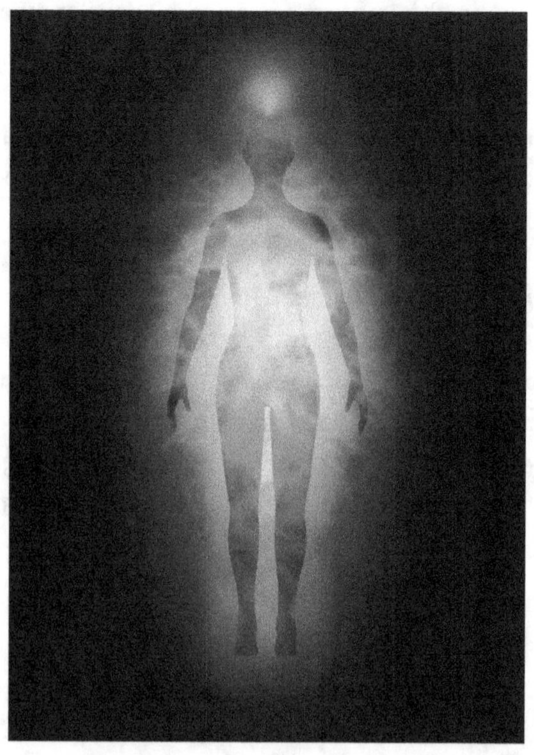

Boosting energy in developmental processes will guide you to self-healing. The benefits of efforts you put into achieving your goal will prove rewarding. In addition, you will find it easier to maintain your body and mind. Some of the popular methods in boosting energy for self-healing are to meditate.

Meditation will guide your mind to learn, develop new ideas, etc. which helps to relieve stress. Stress causes many health problems when it gets out of control. Learn the many different meditation skills to improve your life for living a happier and healthier, longer life. Meditation has come to be one of the most effective ways to improve and maintain health today. More and more people are practicing meditation for energy development and self-healing.

Self-development changes, since we all learn to meditate in our own way. What may work for some people may not work for you. The key is finding what works best for you. Writing for Self-Healing

Writing is a form of meditation. This is because writing helps you to set, and reach goals. When you write you discover your inner needs, self and more. This guides you to explore, which is a form of meditation. Knowing who you are and how you really feel about things you do, can guide you to self-healing. When you discover and learn from your mistakes, it will help give you an energy boost by making changes.

By writing your goals and reaching them brings things to life so you can go back and see for yourself just how far you go to success. When you read your goals and the success, you made it can help you to be more energetic and happier with the results of your efforts. Some people think they have to meditate with their eyes closed. This is not so because when we write we are meditating by focusing on what to write. In addition, we focus on our feelings and thoughts, which help us to come closer to knowing who we are.

This brings us many benefits. We can use meditation to make better decisions. Making better decisions requires that you make necessary changes to reform your way of thinking and the way you live your life. Some people may think that meditation requires closing your eyes however this is not true, since when you right you use deep concentration practices to bring the mind to focus. When you first attempt to focus, your mind will try to toss in interferences. This is because your mind is battling the stress of the day. Let these thoughts go so that you can concentrate shortly with fewer interruptions.

Allowing the thoughts in will relieve stress so that it takes a hike and you can focus more readily. Sometimes you have to look back at your day, or the memories that is making you uneasy. This is the process of healing the mind. Let it go. Keep in mind that what you have no control of will only kill you if you continue to worry. Let it go so that you learn to change only the things you have control of, which each stressor you let go helps you to heal the mind and body.

Take time to analyze. This will help you clear your mind so that you can remove those interferences. Refocus so that you can return to writing. This will help you battle negative thoughts, which clears the mind. You make better choices with a clear mind.

Chapter 6 - Training the Mind to Think Right

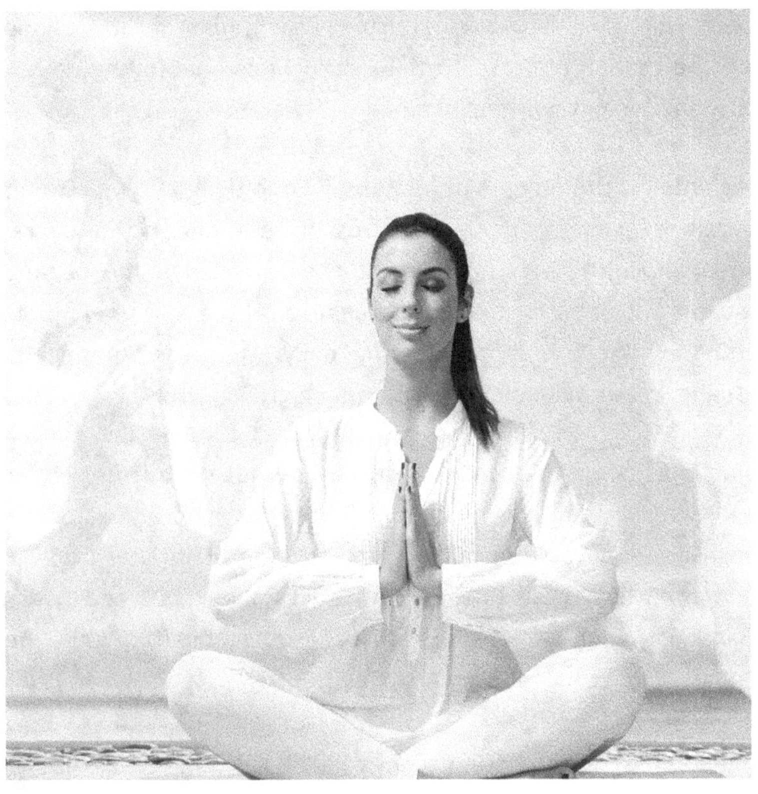

Thinking straight is the key to making good decisions on how we feel about the way we live and perform our lives. We all need to learn to practice meditation in energy development and self-healing by thinking straight to perform and be more successful. When we are thinking of many things all at once, we often become confused. Yet when we learn to focus on one thing at a time, when it comes to making decision to be successful we often succeed. When the mind is clear of chaos, it often helps us to see the steps we need to take to achieve our goals. We also see what we need to maintain our health. To be happy and proud of ourselves we need to know who we are in the first place.

Meditation helps you to find yourself and to decide if you are happy with your current situation. Are there changes you can make to relieve stress for success? Using your thinking straight attitude ask yourself what can you do to change things in order to be happy with the outcome. Learn to think straight by meditating daily to boost energy and self-healing.

Meditation is the process of focusing on one thing at a time to find success. Negative thoughts and stress have a tendency to distract us from focusing on one thing at a time. Change the negative thoughts and stress to thinking straight to relieve that stress that is getting in the way by meditating daily. We program negative thoughts in our mind all the while we are growing up.

Sometimes people say things like, you cannot do this or why are you trying it that way, you failed once why do it again? The negative influences trap in our mind and the brain later brings to the front what these negative influences said to us and uses it against us. When we least expect it these negative thoughts, they jump in to make us think we are a failure.

Overcome the negative thoughts by telling yourself repeatedly that you are going to make changes. Using self-talk practices and meditation, tell yourself that success is just around the corner. By focusing on positive thoughts, it will help you to reach success. Using meditation by focusing on how to overcome the negative thoughts will reprogram the brain and mind to relieve unwanted stress. Stress is the major cause for us to feel like a failure in life. When we feel like we failed, it makes us want to give up and we start letting depression in. Learning meditation in energy development and self-healing with thinking straight will help relieve stress before it tries to take over.

Be in control of your feelings and success by thinking straight. You can practice each day to retrain your mind. As you relieve stress and learn to focus with meditation, you will soon notice small changes. Your energy will increase. Having energy will help you to focus on becoming healthier. Possibly, you may join an exercise class to lose all that weight gain from feeling depressed and absorbing in lazy practices due to no energy. Walking will help to relieve stress as well as limber up your joints that became stiff from not having the energy to do anything.

Exercise is good for everyone to gain control of ourselves to be healthier and happier. Today is a good time to start feeling better and gain control with meditation in energy development and self-healing with thinking straight. Thinking straight by focusing will help you reach your goals successfully. It's time to take back your success by boosting energy for self-healing.

Chapter 7- How to Harness the Powers of Meditation

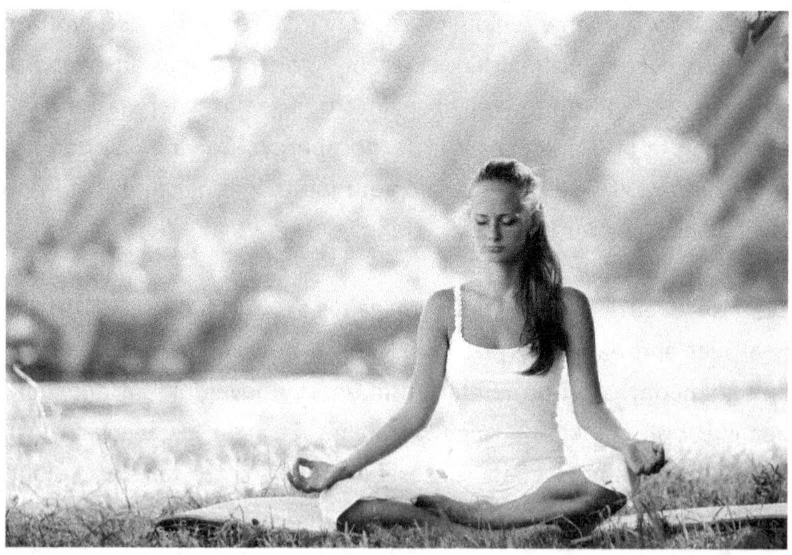

In order to become successful we need positive energy. When we lack energy, we feel hopeless. Sometimes we have to take steps to rebuild the energy loss. To do this however, we just have to find what works best for us. When we feel stress, and our energy is weak, we become down in the dumps and unhappy. Our diet gets out of control and often we fail to exercise. At the workplace, our performance starts to drop to the floor.

Depression will set in and take over if we don't learn how to become in control with how we feel about ourselves. All of this negative noise causes us to become unsuccessful. Take control now and learn the skills and techniques of meditation for energy development in self-healing to reach your success. Meditation is a brain exercise that helps you to develop new skills by conjuring up new ideas that will guide you to success.

Start today by taking over your life and learning to practice meditation for self-development and self-healing. By learning to think positive and finding out who you are success will come to you. You can reprogram your brain and mind to think positive to make changes and build energy development in self-healing. Your brain needs to learn to refocus those negative energies that came alive in your brain from your past. For instance, if someone had said that, you can't play basketball, or you can't walk that far.

These are negative thoughts that the brain heard and it stores them for use later. That little voice in the back of your head pops up saying negative things, repeating what all those negative influences said to you in the past.

By creating a list of goals, you gain advantages. You can use your list to reprogram your mind to think positive by setting a workable plan. Read the list over many times a day until you drive the message home. Repeating the list will eventually help you overcome the negative thoughts and soon these thoughts will begin to think positive. After repeating the list a few times, you will soon begin to show your positive thinking through your self-confidence that you develop from making better decisions. You will have more energy, and smiles will be more frequent. When you feel happy and smile more often, you find it easier to get through the roughest days.

Take some time each day for you. Learn to guide your mind to success by focusing on what it takes to make your life healthier and happier. When you start to feel better and like whom you are, it will help you reach that rainbow at the end of your road. Soon energy will increase, which you will notice an amazing difference. You will feel surprised at the changes that will follow once you boost energy and work toward self-healing.

Energy development will relieve stress that has been building up inside that made you feel depressed and down in the dumps. As the energy builds higher, your self-healing techniques will kick in to help you make better decision so you won't be in the dumps so often. Using certain practices that work for you will encourage you to take care of you by focusing on a healthier living. You will make better decisions with a diet plan that helps you lose weight you gained during the, down in the dumps period.

Start an exercise program to get you out and enjoy life to become healthier and happier. Get to writing so you can boost energy and work toward self-healing successfully.

Forms of Self-Healing Meditation

Tai Chi & Yoga

Tai Chi is a very gentle form of exercise that anyone can do. Since most people spend most of their time sitting, it is imperative that regular exercise become a part of their daily routine. Tai Chi can become that daily movement.

Exercise helps by improving circulatory function, reducing headache tension, lowering blood pressure, and eliminating chronic back and neck pain.

Tai Chi is a series of movements and stretches that anyone can do from any position, even sitting. The exercise will improve posture, stamina, and flexibility.

Movements in Tai Chi are slow and deliberate, and easy to learn. Attending a class is the best way to learn Tai Chi. Do not worry about not being in shape; Tai Chi is known to be an exercise that is done by all types of people, of all ages.

Yoga

Yoga is a great exercise activity for all types of people. It is not difficult, but you do have to want to learn about it. The main goal of yoga is to create a balanced relationship between you physical and mental health.

Yoga is a way of life that is carried throughout the day, not just while in yoga class. Yoga creates an awareness of yourself and your day to day life. This is a drastic change to many people who often live on autopilot.

You can decide how you want to use yoga, for its basic purpose of bringing together mind and body, or as more of a strenuous activity for exercise purposes.

In yoga, it is best to start out at the lowest level possible and work your way up as you develop strength and understanding. Just like most other things, it is important to know the foundational concepts before branching out into more difficult territory,

You can take instructor-led classes, or learn at home through the wide variety of DVDs.

Birkram Yoga

Birkram yoga is also known as "hot yoga", mainly because it is practiced in a space that has been heated to over 115 degrees. Hot yoga mainly focuses on stretches and balance. It also is filled with moves that create pressure in the body that blocks circulation. By going through the movements, the constant buildup of pressure created by stretching are then released, providing a rush of blood through the veins. This is believed to clean them out.

There are 26 poses in hot yoga. The purpose for the hot environment in Birkram yoga is the warmth warms the body's muscles and tendons which aids in flexibility.

There are a few tips for people considering this type of yoga. First, because it is practiced in a hot room, you will sweat a lot. It is best to wear appropriate light clothing. It is also a good idea to drink plenty of water prior to your session.

Hatha Yoga

The main focus of Hatha yoga is breathing, meditation, and posture. The practice of this form of yoga is perfect for people that are new to it. Hatha yoga has more of a strong emphasis on the mental component of meditation, mixed in with yoga.

Karma Yoga

The Karma form of yoga pulls together the spiritual and physical worlds. The fundamentals of Karma yoga are based in the Hindu philosophy and religion. It combines two competing philosophies in the world; from the West – that life should be pleasure based, and from the East – that life should be lived for knowledge. Both theories are blended in karma.

Your karma growth is dependent on how you live your life. Bad karma comes from living your life for the purpose of money, wealth, and material possessions. Good karma comes from living your life for happiness and love.

Karma yoga helps you focus on your life as you learn about your life goals, and helps guide you in the right direction.

CHAPTER 8- TREATMENT PLANS THAT YOU CAN USE

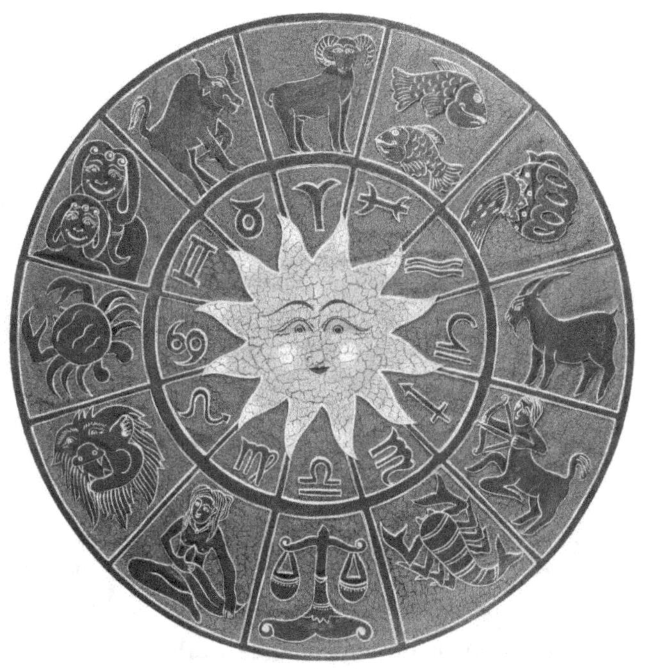

Mind and body are easily defined, but what is the "spirit" of you? The spirit, or soul, can be considered the part of you that is spiritually passionate. What makes you passionate? Here are a few ideas that can help you decide:

1. Look forward to something that you can anticipate.

2. Create a happy place where you can go when you meditate.

3. Reminisce about your successes.

4. Find something that relieves your stress and do it.

5. Explore your future goals – not money related.

Kama-Sutra

The Kama-Sutra is ancient text about sexual health that was written sometime between the 1st and 6th century in India. There are 35 chapters that cover everything from how to find a wife, to how to perform in bed, to how to make you attractive to others.

Sections of the book cover the relationship between diet and sexual wellbeing. Wholesome, nutritious foods are specifically referenced. Histamines are recommended, through food, for increased sexual pleasure.

Breathing techniques are stressed. This helps ease stress and improves overall sexual health.

Feng Shui

Feng Shui is the concept of bring nature and natural patterns and surroundings into our homes and everyday lives. This will bring harmony and peaceful alignment with the world.

Feng Shui brings together all of the elements. Fire, earth, air, and water, and the additional "metal", are represented inside the home by the selection of lighting, scents, sounds, and the placement of furniture and fixtures.

The underlying concept is that the qi, or life force, must be able to move freely in a room. Therefore, the location of furniture, for example, is important.

Chiropractic

Chiropractic is an alternative medicinal practice that is now considered conventional. The main theory behind chiropractic is that the vertebrate of the spine is not in alignment. It is believed that this misalignment causes many diseases and disorders throughout the body.

Chiropractors use pressure to realign and adjust the spine. Most chiropractors also look at the whole picture – stress, lifestyle choices, and overall health – when recommending treatment.

Chiropractors have been known to heal a wide range of medical problems through their work on patient's backs. Asthma, migraines, arthritis and more issues can all be positively impacted.

This treatment is safe and usually inexpensive. It is non-evasive. Going to a chiropractor will certainly require regular visits because your issues will not be fully treated in just one session.

Chapter 9 - Does Alternative Medicine Work on Children?

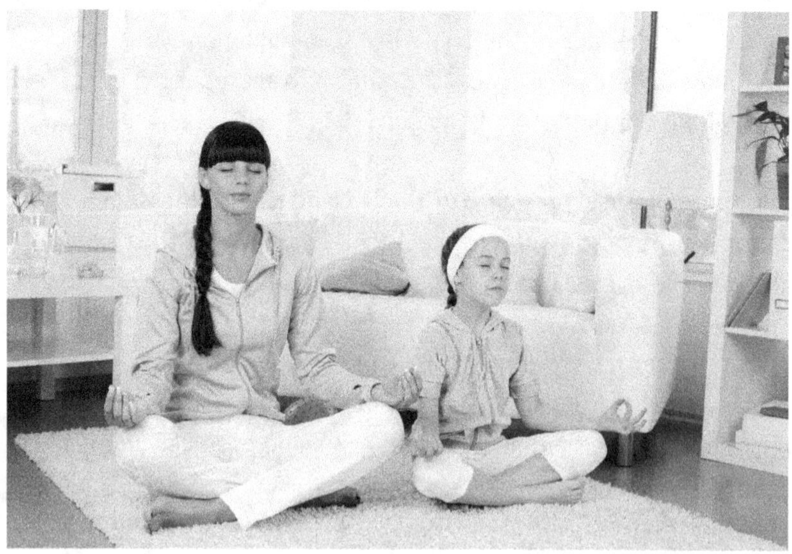

Sometimes conventional treatments are not an option for children. One example of when alternative medicines are a viable option for children is when they refuse to take their over-the-counter medication. They might be more willing to take an herbal remedy because it is something different.

Consider discussing with your conventional doctor these supplementary treatments for children:

Acupuncture

The needles release endorphins to the brain which can help kids with asthma, and reduce other pains.

Hypnosis

This technique might give a child more discipline regarding the regular administration of their conventional medication.

Relaxation techniques and massage

This can help kids with asthma deal with constricting airways. Massage can help relax the stress surround asthma as well. Breathing techniques can help kids feel in control of their breathing. Kids with more serious diseases such as diabetes and cancer can use the relaxing benefits of massage to relieve stress and help maintain a positive outlook.

Always do plenty of research and consult with your child's doctor before beginning any alternative medical techniques.

Of Gender and Alternative Medicine

Men and women each have their own medical needs specific to their gender. It is wise to consider what areas of alternative medicine are best geared for your gender.

For women, issues related to menstruation – such as regular menstruation and PMS are always hot topics. For these issues, women have the following homeopathic options:

Acupuncture

Chinese medicinal herbs & herbal teas

Osteopathy

Crystal therapy

Yoga

Hypnosis

For men, issues around prostate health and overall wellbeing can involve an alternative approach. Men have these choices:

Yoga

Acupuncture

Herbal treatments

Men and women both need to care for their health. A proactive, homeopathic approach will ensure a happy, healthy life.

Chapter 10 - Treating Serious Ailments through Alternative Care

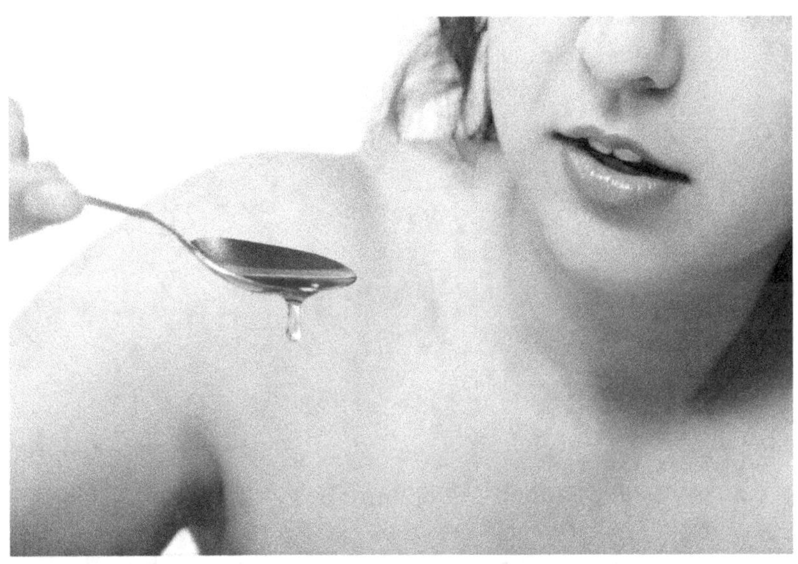

Obesity

There are alternative techniques that can be used in the fight to lose unwanted pounds. Of course, just like in conventional medicine, there is no magic pill. However, the standard "eat well, be more active" technique of losing weight can be enhanced with alternative medicine.

First, you can consider yoga. This exercise is slow and calculated, but the results can be dramatic. When practices wholeheartedly and regularly, you can gain muscle and lose fat.

Acupuncture can reduce food cravings that are sabotaging your weight loss efforts. Teas can help curb cravings as well as detoxify the body.

Self-Diagnosis, Healing and Recovery
Follow these tips to lose weight with alternative medicine:

1. Use a juicer to drink your fruits and vegetables.

2. Add Omega-3 to your beverages.

3. Visit a homeopathic doctor for a nutritional evaluation.

4. Contact an herbalist for recommendations on alternative teas.

5. Consider taking bovine or shark cartilage.

6. Hypnosis can be used for behavioral modification.

Cancer

People with cancer often look for viable options that they can use to fight this disease. Unfortunately, there is no cure for cancer. Conventional treatments are the most aggressive, and while alternative and conventional medicine should work together to provide a comprehensive medical experience, at this time they do not.

You can use alternative medicine to supplement your conventional cancer treatments. Here are some of the best complementary alternative treatments:

1. Acupuncture: Helps with nausea, tiredness, pain, headaches.

2. Herbal remedies: Ginger, for one, is helpful in dealing with nausea and vomiting caused by chemotherapy.

3. Hyperbaric oxygen therapy is currently being studies as a complementary treatment for radiation therapy.

4. Massage helps relieve fatigue.

One of the biggest benefits of complimentary treatments is that the sick person can take control over their situation and treatment, even if just in a small way. This helps the patient's chances for survival and improves the quality of life.

As with any medical treatment, consult with your doctor before self-treating. Dangerous and counterproductive side effects can result if treatment is not cohesively planned.

What Happens in an Alternative Treatment Session?

First and foremost, it is essential to pick the right practitioner for you. When selecting your perfect practitioner, be sure to review their credentials because there are many fraudulent practitioners in the alternative medical world.

Follow these tips to find the perfect practitioner:

1. Search the phone book and online for local professionals. Select a local group of practitioners.

2. Research this group of practitioners to find out their experience, education, style, and anything else you can about them.

3. Find out what organizations they are affiliated with. The more trade groups, the better.

4. Contact them to ask what specific experience they have with your type of situation.

5. Ask what the treatment process is for your given situation.

Self-Diagnosis, Healing and Recovery

The focus of an alternative medicine session is different then what occurs in a conventional medical session. Here, the practitioner will want to learn about you as a whole person, not just the specific area of injury or concern.

How to Become an Alternative Medical Practitioner

Are you thinking about becoming an alternative medical practitioner? The profession is rewarding and interesting, and provides you with the opportunity to help people. By providing an alternative medicine service, you will be making a difference in the world.

First, you will need to determine which type of alternative medicine you want to practice. Alternative medicine is broken down into seven categories:

1. Dioelectricmagnetic applications

2. Diet

3. Nutrition

4. Lifestyle changes

5. Herbal medicine

6. Manual healing

7. Biological treatments

To become a professional alternative medicine practitioner, you will need to successfully complete an accredited program at a registered school. There are many schools that specialize in one area or another of alternative medicine.

Schooling is intensive, and a good program will include years of study and practice, as well as an internship experience.

Once you have completed school and practicum work you will be able to practice your field of study on your own.

Paying for Alternative Medicine

Prices for alternative treatments vary. Most treatments are not covered by insurance, so it is important to discuss actual costs prior to receiving services from a practitioner.

The first step in finding out how to pay for treatment is to call your insurance company to see if they will cover your treatment session. If they do cover, find out the specifics. How many sessions? Is there a specific type of treatment that is only covered?

When you meet your practitioner, one of the first questions to ask is if they accept your type of insurance. If you are not using insurance, you will need to work out alternative payment.

CHAPTER 11- TOOLS FOR ENERGY DEVELOPMENT AND SELF-HEALING

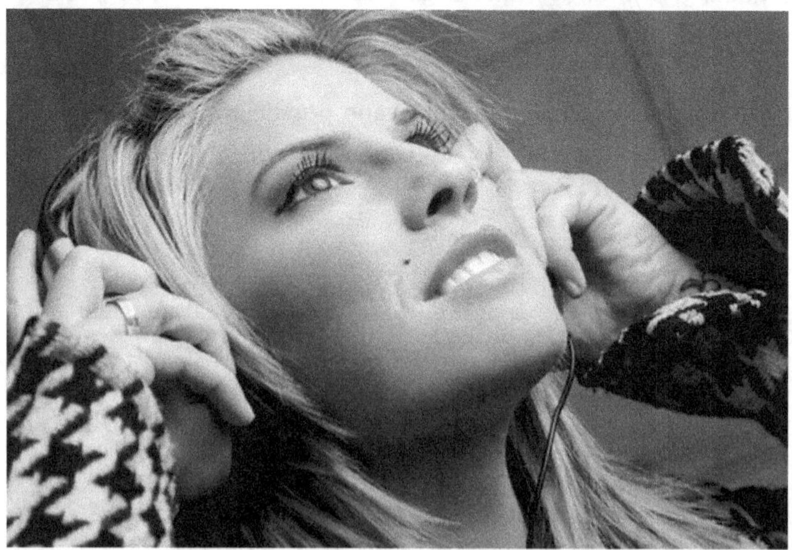

There is always time and room for gaining new skills for energy development and self-healing. With the world turning and moving in technology so fast anymore that daily stress is impossible to avoid. Everyone has stress that cannot be avoided on a daily basis's but then there is the pop up stress, when we least expect it. For instance making decision on whether you take time to exercise or run someone to the doctor. You may get a disturbing letter in the mail that causes you to worry and get angry. We can use these stressors to learn how to control stress.

As we grow older, meditation skills are necessary. When we are small, many stressful things happen but we do not realize what is going on so it doesn't make us angry or scared. As an adult, we have to learn how to handle stressful things and make decisions on how to handle them. Stress can cause many things to a person causing them to perform less, lose energy, chronic pain and even diseases like depression can set in. We can learn to control our feelings and handle stress making it easier to make good decisions.

Meditating will help relieve the unneeded stress that is the most common cause for many illnesses. Use the tools below to learn how to feel better about you. Let these tools guide you to making better decisions. Practice meditation anytime and anywhere by focusing on what you're doing. Tools:

Goals

We all need goals in life to keep us active and healthy. If we don't feel good about ourselves, why be successful? Using your positive thinking tool will help you to see yourself in full light. You can use this tool to set goals and to see where you want to go in life. You need to be honest and truthful when looking at yourself in order to make good decisions on how you want to be a success for the future.

Do you like the way you look and feel? Are you happy with your workplace? Are there things in your life that don't really need to be there? Are you happy with your relationship? Write your feelings down to make them a part of your life. Now look inside and make decisions on how you can make good decisions to eliminate them.

Turn these unwanted stressful items into joy. Write down how you can change these things to make them good thoughts. Write your goals. Reread what you write daily as a reminder to grow. When you begin to think negative things about how you feel, reading your goals will remind you to think positive in the changes you working on.

Music

You can use music to help relieve stress. Many people have different kinds of music that will help them sleep and relax. It doesn't matter what music you listen to; maybe a fast beat is what it takes to give you energy. Turn it up to get your house cleaned. If you're a person that like's soft and slow music to relax with when you go to bed at night; put the CD player on low to help you sleep more restful. You have many options with relaxing music tools today. The different music gives you options that guide you to relaxation.

Try them out by getting on the Internet and downloading them on your PC to listen to when working or playing. Some of these downloads are free just for trying them. For more information on how to meditate for energy development and self-healing, search the Internet or at your local library, you'll be glad you decided to learn the skills and the practice of meditation for energy development and self-healing. Use your brainwork tools to achieve your goals.

Brainwork Tools

When you need that fire rise in self-healing, you must find the time to explore your mind and find your inner intelligence. Since, our new age is moving toward technology, which requires that we learn some new ways to stay healthy and cope with the increasing stress. We all deal with stress each day that comes from stressors that mount up.

Overwhelming stress can lead to trouble, so the first thing we need to do is find a way to manage stress. We all have received a disturbing letter in the mail that affords you to feel stress that sometimes makes you angry. We can use forthwith stressors to learn how to control the pressure rather than allowing it to weigh us down. As we start the generative process, we have to learn how to handle stress. So take the driver's seat and learn how to handle the pressure that weighs you down. You want to manage stress, simply because we are in a state of war, as well as driven toward learning technology at advanced states.

Violence is common in our world. We live around this pressure in our neighborhoods, and in our world. Sometimes the stressors cause us to perform less, blow up, punch walls, feel chronic hurt and even diseases like woefulness can set in. We can learn to control our circle and handle stress, making it easier on the body and mind. Some of the best practices that can benefit us in many ways, including meditation,

Meditating will support your mind and body and help to relieve the unnecessary stress. You want to make this a habit each day, since stress when it takes control can lead to fatal diseases and even death. Use your tools beneath your mind to learn how to improve your health by taking control of your stress. Consider subliminal training as a guide to use your inner tools. Let your inner tools direct you to making better decisions. Iterate imagination anytime and anywhere by focusing on what you want from life. Let your visualizations lead you to your dreams and invoke you to take action.

Additional Tools that You Can Use

Values

We all need goals in extent to keep us active and healthy. If we don't feel good about ourselves, we often fail success. Exploring and developing your positive thinking tools will assist you by helping you in half model reshaping. You can use innate tool to set goals. Use these tools to create workable plans to achieve your goals. You need to be honest and truthful intermittently looking inside you in order to develop energy for self-healing. Search inside you and sit in the saddle, learning how you can make wise decisions to eliminate problems that hinder your health. Direct these unwanted grievous issues to joy.

Write down how you can change straightaway things to create good thoughts. Write your ethics down. Check through what you have written, using it as a keepsake to grow. When you start to dwell on balky things, read your list and use it as something to remind you of your goals. You want to train your body and mind to relax.

Relaxation is necessary to cut back on risks of heart disease or other common diseases related to stress. You have options if you find it difficult to take the load of self-healing alone. You have natural medicines, musical relaxation options, subliminal training, Neurofeedback, and more, just search the net or visit your local library. You will feel amazed at the helpful guides that will lead you to energy development and self-healing. Give that brain a good workout.

Chapter 12- How to Develop Positive Thinking and Better Decision Making

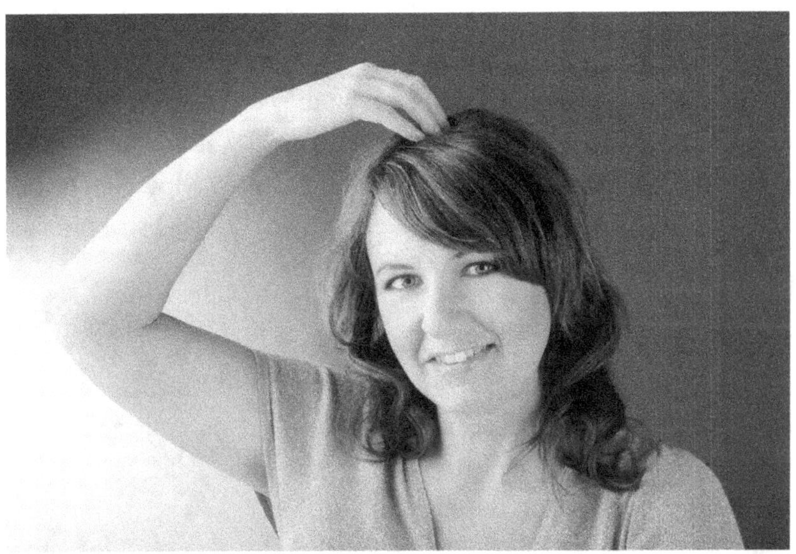

Thinking Positive in meditation will give you a boost of energy for self-healing. By learning new skills on making changes with a positive attitude, you will begin to show signs of feeling better about yourself and success. Dig down and bring out your inner feelings about how you feel with the success you have accomplished.

Do you feel happy with your career? Do you feel content with how you live? Do you like how you look? How about your health, are you content with your current health? Now, think positive and write these feelings on paper.

Once you have put your true feelings on paper they will be more realistic to help you think positive on making changes to be where you really want to be. By thinking positive, you will make better decisions. You will see the changes you need to make successfully complete your goals. Take control of your life by thinking positive to give yourself a boost to make better decisions. When we don't feel good about ourselves, we feel stressed and make poor decisions.

Relieve that stress to make better decisions before depression takes control. Learn to relieve stress to give you relaxation for better decision-making, more energy and living happier. When we feel stressed, the stress often causes us to develop many health problems. We often feel pain and lose sleep. Without sleep, we wake up tired and decisions are harder to make because we focus on how tired we are instead of the decision itself.

You can learn to relieve stress by making goals to have a better life with success when thinking positive in meditating for energy development and self-healing. Once you've made your goals and decided how you're going to change learn the skills of thinking positive and focusing on the changes.

When we focus and practice thinking positive we are learning the meditation skills as well. Reprogram your brain and mind to think positive by focusing and repeating the list of changes often. Some people think once a day reading the list is enough. Wrong, the more you read the list the better. Repeating it many times a day whenever you begin to think negative will help reprogram the brain to override the negative thoughts to positive ones. As you reprogram your mind, it makes the stress become less, because your confidence will build to help you with making better decisions.

Thinking positive by learning to make better decisions will help you relieve stress, since you will learn how to eliminate stressors. Relieve unwanted stress by thinking positive will also help you increase your energy development skills. Soon you will have more energy than you know what to do with. Use up some of this energy by exercising the brain as well as your body. Everyone's brain needs to have exercise just like the body. When we exercise the brain, it helps to prevent aging, which encourages a longer and healthier life. Learn to exercise the brain by using your positive thinking tools.

Encouraging the brain to think positive and making better decisions helps us to stay younger and keep our memory from fading as we age. Keeping your brain and mind active will give it the exercise it needs to help us exercise the body. Our body needs to stay strong and healthy to living longer. As we age, our bodies become stiff, sore, and useless. With exercise you can keep, your body stronger and healthier to relieve pain and stress that causes so many of us to become depressed.

Stay in control of your brain and mind with exercise to staying healthier as well as happy. Begin thinking positive in meditation for energy development and self-healing to become the person you really want to be. Develop your accepted efficacious wisdom now to develop energy in self-healing.

Accepted Efficacious

When you develop accepted efficacious wisdom in energy development and positive self-healing, you learn to think positive by making better decisions. A sound mind takes you into speculation and directs you to give you the energy boost for self-healing. When you think positive, you start to develop new skills on regulatory changes, which results in a positive attitude.

Develop Positive Thinking

Learning to think positive requires meditation. You need to focus on your past learning to find ways to develop new skills. Focus on what your accomplishments. Draw from these accomplishments by considering your life now. Write down your feelings, thoughts and so on to use them to your advantage as you work on your goal to develop energy for self-healing. Review what you write. Use the new learning to your advantage by dwelling on your accomplishments and focusing on what you did to achieve. By Pondering over progressive learning, you will learn to choose options better that lead you to build energy.

With the new learning, you should see ways to successfully blanket, making changes to achieve your goals. Learn to take charge of your existence developing new skills to give you advancement so you can get in the saddle. For now, our mission is to reduce stress. However, stress can work in your advantage, so learn how to use stress as a tool to take control of your life. Learn how to dull stress so you guide your mind and body to relaxation. When you feel strained, the pressure habitually sets us up to soup up many health care problems. We begin to feel stress because we do not receive proper rest.

We have the power to learn how to relieve the impact of stress by examining our life. We can learn to make better life choices by fluctuating and pondering over positive ways to connect with our inner being. This comes from meditating for liveliness development and self-healing. On and off, we strive toward practicing thinking accepted efficacious wisdom and when we are literature, we feel lively.

Learn to program your gray matter differently so you can analyze positive learning by focusing on your goals and repeating actions needed to reach your aim. The more effort you put in to learning the more you construe. Recurring stress becomes larger in a day whenever you originate to study negative thoughts rather than reprogram the brain to circumvent the negative thoughts. Once you learn to reprogram your thinking, stress disappears and reappears presenting itself as a reward rather than a negative force. You will notice energy increase at this point.

Develop a positive mind by erudition to make helpful choices will assist you with reducing negative pressures. You will learn to blot out stressors, rather than allow them to accumulate and cause unwelcoming stress that causes you harm. Not long after you progress, you affect to have developed energy or power than your body and mind can sustain. You move to exit some of this get-up-and-go juice by exerting the encephalon in addition to the body. Alternately, when we exert the cerebrum, it aids us with the prevention of progressive aging. It succors us in to living longer. Welcome the intelligence to conceive positive and regulatory thinking. Learn to relax to encourage youth and to retain your memory to slow fermenting aging.

Learn to develop your accepted efficacious wisdom to develop energy for self-healing. Each day you practice, the load lightens, which puts you in the saddle and in control of the reigns.

About the Author

Allison McPhee was born in India to missionary parents. She has spent her first few years exploring the Indian countryside and falling in love with the culture and tradition.

When she was 15, her family moved back to the US but she brought with her her passion for Hindu culture. She does yoga and is often seen meditating. Her ability to be at peace with herself is the key to her composure and ethereal calmness.

9 781681 275208